Eczema Remedies

How to Relieve Eczema

With Diet & Natural Remedies

Natalie J. Stevens

While every precaution has been taken in the preparation of this book, the publisher assumes no responsibility for errors or omissions, or for damages resulting from the use of the information contained herein.

ECZEMA REMEDIES

HOW TO RELIEVE ECZEMA

WITH DIET & NATURAL REMEDIES

First edition. May 19, 2021.

Written by Natalie J. Stevens.

TABLE OF CONTENTS

Introduction

What exactly is eczema? Eczema is a spectrum of skin disorders that includes atopic dermatitis, touch dermatitis, dyshidrotic eczema, hand eczema, neurodermatitis, nummular eczema, stasis dermatitis, and stasis dermatitis. Finding a natural eczema remedy that is both calming and effective can be life-changing for those who suffer from this bothersome disease. This is how skin rashes and autoimmune disorders are represented. Dryness typically occurs on the wrists, elbows, feet, knees, and face. When scratched, rashes on infected areas begin to itch and become more inflamed. This disease is not contagious, but it does last a long time.

Furthermore, the strength of it can change over time. Some children will outgrow their allergies, while others will continue to be extremely vulnerable. Additional illnesses can arise as a result of the current illness. Each patient's symptoms and severity of skin inflammation are unique. Eczema comes in a number of forms. Aside from the most common case, atopic dermatitis, there are about six other disease types, each with its own treatment methods and side effects.

To ensure a clear solution for each case, they should all be established with the aid of a specialist. Atopic dermatitis is the most common form of dermatitis. It's very common in kids, and it's also linked to asthma and hay fever. Action with an allergic material, stress, excessive moisturizing, insect bites, temperature changes, strain, and even genetic predisposition may all cause other forms.

The appearance and side effects of each case are unique. The only thing they have in common is that they are sore and dry skin styles that should not be scratched. When it comes to the origin of eczema, there is no consensus. Various forms of illness are exacerbated by their various beliefs, according to the latest studies. The risk of developing eczema is even greater for children whose parents suffer from the condition.

When both parents are afflicted, the risk multiplies. A long list of external factors may also have an effect on the bodies of susceptible individuals, causing inflammation. There are two kinds of danger sources: internal and external. From the outside, allergenic chemicals, temperature, food, and dust can trigger a skin transformation, while stress and hormonal changes affect symptoms from inside.

Eczema usually occurs in young children, with studies showing that 65 percent of cases appear before a child's first birthday, and 90 percent of those affected have their first case before the age of five. This same study discovered that children who live with a dog are substantially less likely to develop eczema at any age. By the age of three, 39 percent of Caucasian children experience eczema, according to a report conducted by the Department of Pediatrics at Cincinnati Children's Hospital Medical Center.

While eczema outbreaks are most common in infants and young children, it can strike at any age. Although the majority of eczema-related skin disorders are chronic, it's important to remember that contact dermatitis and hand eczema may be acute, resulting from an allergic reaction or chemical exposure.

Eczema is a particular type of skin condition. The source of outbreaks are unique to each individual, as is the location where the rashes occur and the form of rash. Nonetheless, symptoms can be similar in different people, particularly if they are relatives. Itching is the most common symptom, and it can occur in a variety of ways, ranging from mildly irritating to dangerously irritating.

People with eczema have the constant urge to scratch the infected area of skin until it bleeds, which actually worsens the condition. Inflammation of the skin can take several forms. In each case of contact with the unwanted matter, itching and inflammation either go away completely or return. It is strongly advised that you see a local doctor to determine the type of eczema you have and, as a result, treatment options.

The traditional treatment for eczema consists of a series of simple measures aimed at controlling the patient's condition and reducing the impact of disease on the human body. This disease is primarily triggered by an allergic reaction to an external stimulus. As a result, the first step for each person is to determine what is causing their disease and to avoid excessive contact with it. Also, chemicals that are considered to be dermatitis causes should be avoided.

Furthermore, it is important to take special care of yourself, including moisturizing the skin, avoiding stressful conditions, and refraining from scratching. Remedies can also be used to reduce inflammation depending on the condition. Antibiotics are used to prevent people who are suffering from severe skin infections. Antihistamines are used to avoid scratching and to relieve it. Internal and external usage corticosteroid-inclusive medications may be distinguished.

In this situation, external use is strongly recommended, since internal use has a number of negative side effects and can only be used in an emergency. Immunomodulators and wet dressings may also be used to treat some forms of dermatitis. Around the same time, the lack of a remedy provided by traditional medicine prompted society to consider a natural approach to treating this disease. Long-term homeopathy therapy can be more effective in some cases while causing less side effects.

A patient's personality, interests, mental state, and even family problems are all assessed using this method. There are a number of everyday items that can help slow the progression of the disease. Kimchee, rice, soybean meal, and oat are among them. Supplementing the diet with vitamins B, D, and E, as well as eating iodine-rich foods, can be beneficial. Specific bathing ingredients reduce the risk of water-induced inflammation. Probiotics have a positive effect on the disease in certain unusual circumstances.

Aside from that, skin moisturizing is the focus of a number of home-made recipes. Eczema mostly disrupts the skin's self-fattening and self-moistening processes, so different oils should be used to restore the balance. Eczema is incurable. It can, however, be regulated to the point that the symptoms are barely noticeable. There is an inner trigger that makes a disease active in each person; identifying the cause can aid in self-care.

The type of illness is also unique. At the same time, there is no universal agreement on how to care for oneself, since both conventional and natural medicine have their own strengths and weaknesses. Eczema can usually be managed as long as a cause of skin inflammation is not present.

The amount of flare-ups can diminish with age for certain people, and some might even outgrow it completely. Eczema, on the other hand, can come and go throughout one's life. The best course of action is to learn how to handle your eczema and recognize flare-up causes. While there are no known cures for eczema, there are several ways to lessen the intensity of flare ups so that you can lessen your use of medications or eliminate them altogether.

Eczema symptoms can vary from mild to extreme, and they can change from one outbreak to the next. Typical symptoms can look like the following:

- The formation of small, raised bumps that can ooze liquid and form a crust
- Skin that is thick, brittle, scaly and easily cracks
- Infants' hands, feet, ankles, wrists, neck, upper chest, eyelids, skin folds, and face and scalp have red, brown, or grayish patches of skin.
- Scratched sensitive skin that is swollen and raw
- A rash that induces severe itching and disrupts sleep habits and basic daily activities on a regular basis
- Eczema rashes caused by atopic eczema

Eczema Causes, Symptoms, and Risk Factors

Eczema is caused by a variety of factors and has a wide range of risk factors. Furthermore, eczema symptoms vary greatly among those who are affected. Although there is no single cause of eczema, there are a number of factors that contribute to its onset and flare-ups. Furthermore, a diverse set of risk factors has been established.

Some Eczema's Risk Factors Include:

- A hereditary predisposition to eczema, hay fever, or asthma, or a family history of eczema, hay fever, or asthma
- Healthcare workers
- Children who go to daycare

- Children that have ADHD

- Living in a dry environment

- Deficiency in nutrients

- Obesity in adolescents is linked to a later development of eczema

- Low levels of vitamin D during pregnancy may increase the risk of eczema in the first year of life

What are Some Causes of Eczema?

The medical community is also trying to figure out what causes eczema. Some people experience it as a result of a dietary deficiency, while others experience it as a result of an allergen or other irritant. The following are the most commonly known causes of eczema:

- Skin that is dry and responsive and cracks

- Dysfunction of the immune system

- Situational circumstances

- Skin-related gene variations

- Allergies of foods, cosmetics, laundry detergents, and other chemicals

- Stress that lasts a long time
- Changes in temperature

Different Types of Eczema

Are you aware of the type of eczema you have? Eczema comes in a variety of forms, and people who have one type of eczema are more likely to develop another. Here are some of the most common types of eczema.

Atopic Eczema

While you are born with a genetic predisposition to atopic eczema, the environment may also play a role. It's a warning that the immune system is overactive. It is most common in infants, with symptoms appearing in the first few months of life. The vast majority of children will develop out of it by the time they reach puberty. Eczema with atopic dermatitis is becoming more common. AD 15 affects 15% of children in the United States and 7.3% of adults.

In this case, the body produces large amounts of the protein IgE, which is a protein that functions on behalf of the immune system's defensive cells. It triggers allergic reactions in some people. We all have this protein, but people with atopic eczema create a lot more because of their increased sensitivity to certain chemicals, whether by contact, ingestion of certain foods and fluids, or inhalation and breathing airborne particles. The problem is caused by an overactive immune system, which results in skin inflammation. You can develop irritant contact eczema and be predisposed to hay fever and asthma if you have atopic eczema.

House dust mites, also known as bed bugs, pollen, pet fur, skin, and feathers are the most common allergens present in people with atopic eczema. Yeasts present on the body, as well as foods such as cow's milk, soya, wheat, nuts, and eggs, are other allergens. Find out what you're allergic to and stay away from it as far as possible. Get a blood test to help you figure out what's wrong. Dry, sticky, and itchy skin around the neck, knees, wrists, face, and eyelids would be the first signs of flare ups.

Asteatotic Eczema

This is more common in older people, and it usually appears as a red itchy rash on the leg.

Discoid Eczema

Discoid eczema affects people of all ages, but it is more common in older men. Adults have a tendency to overreact to stress and alcohol. It is normal in children and younger people who have a propensity to atopic eczema.

Seborrhoeic Eczema

Adults with large areas of sweat glands on their bodies are more likely to develop this condition. It's caused by an overabundance of pityrosporum, a harmless yeast that forms in the body. It would be beneficial to use an anti-yeast drug.

Because of the greater number of grease glands, it is often found on the scalp, ears, armpits, and groin. The condition can range from mild flaky skin to extreme itching, oiliness, and inflammation of the skin. Anti-yeast shampoos can help to control scalp problems. Coal tar shampoos and selenium shampoos are often used in extreme cases.

Cradle cap on the scalp and folds of the skin are common in babies with this form of eczema. Since their skin is so fragile, you must be certain of the products you use. Emollient creams, antifungal creams, and steroid creams are among the items that are recommended. Hard scaling from cradle cap can be softened with aqueous cream containing salicylic acid. After that, wash your baby's hair with shampoo made specially for babies. Olive oil applied to the scalp is a safe allernativo. This is an old treatment that has been used for many years.

Irritant Contact Eczema

This is a very common occurrence that occurs when someone comes into contact with a material that causes hypersensitivity, accompanied by an allergic reaction as a result of the irritated skin. Many who work in jobs that cause their hands to be wet often, such as hairdressers, restaurant workers, cleaners, those who handle food, nurses, and health workers, are the key groups affected by irritant contact eczema.

This is because we are constantly exposed to such pollutants and chemicals contained in daily items that we use at home and at work. Soap, detergents, and food account for about 85% of the problem. Bleaches, plastic, skin remedies, hairdressing chemicals, and perfumes, as well as paints and many craft-related items such as glues, are all common sources.

Since it is impractical to expect to eliminate all of these issues in the workplace and in daily activities, it is recommended that protective gloves be worn. Since the rubber in most of these gloves will aggravate the condition, you can wear them with cotton inners or purchase a separate pair of lightweight, breathable cotton gloves to wear inside the rubber gloves. This will help to prevent excessive sweating, which can occur while wearing rubber gloves for an extended period of time, which will reduce the risk of an outbreak.

It has the same appearance as regular eczema and is handled similarly to allergic touch eczema. It is important to keep the hands moisturized in order to prevent skin cracking and splitting. Try to find barrier creams that are herbal and chemical-free, as steroid creams have been known to aggravate eczema in certain people.

Allergic Contact Eczema

If you are susceptible to some of these irritant problems, you should have a patch test to identify the potential causes. Certain objects that come into contact with the skin are recognized by the immune system as foreign bodies, and the skin responds to them. Weeping, scratching, and redness on the skin's surface are some of the symptoms. Symptoms usually begin in the immediate area of touch and then spread as the immune cells begin to function.

It's crucial to pay attention to the signs right away so you can figure out what's causing them to stop it in the future. There are things that we use on a daily basis that we are completely unaware of. Here are a couple of them, along with an example of what they're used for:

You should stay away from the following:

- Nickel - used in perfume, jewelry, studs on trousers, bra clips, and butterfly earring backs
- Plants - allergic responses to touch and breathing, similar to hay fever
- Rubber - some of our clothes and shoes contain rubber and other chemicals, which you may not be aware of
- Epoxy resins - also known as hobby craft adhesives, are a form of epoxy resin
- Colophony - used in plasters
- Paraphenylenediamine - used in some henna products and black hair dyes
- Potassium dichromate - used in leather goods
- Emollient creams of cetearyl alcohol

- Neomycin is an antibiotic. Fusidic acid is a type of antibiotic. steroid creams containing hydrocortisone lanolin – a moisturizer

The Importance of Diet When Dealing with Eczema

Some foods can cause the release of T cells, which cause inflammation, as well as immunoglobulin-E, or IgE, an antibody produced by the body in response to a threat. Nuts, milk, and wheat are all foods that cause inflammation.

Eating such foods can cause the body to release immune system compounds that cause inflammation, which leads to an eczema flare-up in people with eczema. A diet that is anti-eczema is similar to a diet that is anti-inflammatory.

Certain foods may not tend to cause eczema, but they can cause a flare-up if you already have the disease. Maintaining an eczema-friendly diet is important for long-term eczema treatment. Not everyone will respond to the same foods in the same way or experience the same flare-ups.

Your dermatitis can be significantly improved if you follow an elimination diet, which includes removing certain foods one by one. This will help you figure out which foods are causing your eczema. This can be performed under the supervision of your doctor or a nutritional therapist, or on your own. However, if you work with someone, they will advise you on appropriate alternative foods to ensure that you are not deficient in any essential nutrients.

The foods that will be discussed contain properties that can help reduce eczema flare-ups, but it's important to get to know your body and what foods work best for you.

Basic Guidelines for an Anti-Inflammatory Diet

The key factor in how you eat is to make sure you are consuming anti-inflammatory foods. This is how you can help to alleviate or minimize the symptoms of eczema. Since inflammation is a crucial part of eczema, eating an anti-inflammatory is extremely important. Elevated insulin levels result from high-sugar and refined-carbohydrate diets, which encourage inflammation.

Instead, focus on whole grain carbs, protein, and a variety of vegetables.

Getting the right mix of fats in your diet (especially those high in omega-3) can also help to reduce inflammation.

If you don't have any allergies, eating a lot of oily fish, meat, nuts, grains, and flax oil may be helpful.

Foods to Avoid

It is highly recommended to avoid these foods entirely, in order to avoid flare ups:

- Eggs
- Soy products
- Cow's milk
- Gluten
- Nuts

Preservatives and artificial additives in foods can worsen symptoms. Foods rich in trans fats, such as margarine, processed foods, and fast food, fall into this category.

Sugary foods can also negatively affect eczema flare-ups. Sugar triggers an increase in insulin levels, which can lead to inflammation.

Sugar is commonly found in the following foods:

- Various coffee beverages
- Sugary sodas
- Sugary juices
- Smoothies
- Desserts
- Burgers
- Various fast food items
- Sugary snacks
- Various condiments

So What Foods Should You Eat?

Foods That Contain Quercetin

Foods containing quercetin are very important. Quercetin is a flavonoid found in plants. It is what contributes to the vibrant color of many flowers, fruits, and vegetables.

It's both an antihistamine and an antioxidant. This means it will lower inflammation and histamine levels in your body.

Which foods are high in quercetin?

- Kale
- Broccoli
- Spinach
- Cherries
- Blueberries
- Apples

Fatty fish, such as salmon and herring, can help to alleviate your symptoms. Omega-3 fatty acids, which are anti-inflammatory, are abundant in fish oil.

You may also want to look at taking an omega-3 supplement. In general, consuming at least 250 mg of omega-3 fatty acids every day, preferably via food, is recommended.

Probiotics

Live cultures in probiotic foods, such as yogurt, help build a healthy immune system. This can aid in the reduction of allergic reactions or flare-ups. You can also take a probiotic supplement, which can be very beneficial in relieving eczema systems, as well as benefit your overall health. Taking a high-quality probiotic supplement of 24–100 billion species daily should be considered during an eczema occurrence and to eliminate significant flares.

Foods high in probiotics include:

- Unpasteurized sauerkraut
- Naturally fermented pickles
- Kefir
- Soft cheeses
- Tempeh
- Sourdough bread
- Miso soup

Keep in mind, your best foods are usually determined by any food allergies you might have. Foods that are considered eczema-friendly can cause an allergic reaction in those who are allergic to them.

Vitamin C-rich foods may help minimize absorption of these components.

A diet rich in fresh fruits and vegetables can also be beneficial. This contains the following:

- Mango
- Pineapple
- Oranges
- Strawberries
- Cauliflower
- Kale

Benefits of Avoiding Gluten-Containing Foods?

Celiac disorder and eczema appear to go side by side for some people. This may be due to the fact that both diseases share a genetic connection. Gluten is removed from the diet to treat Celiac disease. If you have celiac disease or gluten sensitivity in addition to eczema, eliminating gluten can help your skin look better.

Gluten-free food has gained prominence, and many foods now bear the gluten-free logo. Gluten-free alternatives are available for most wheat, rye, and barley goods. Here, a little creativity goes a long way. For example, instead of bread crumbs, potato flakes can be used to coat chicken cutlets, and almond flour can be used instead of wheat flour when baking.

Flavonoids have anti-eczema properties

According to new findings, flavonoids (chemicals contained in fruits and vegetables) and polyphenols (chemicals found in plants) can be useful to people with eczema. They have a variety of health effects, but they tend to improve in this case by lowering histamine levels and improving the skin's capacity to resist infection. Many different flavonoids have been studied in this field, but quercetin appears to be particularly successful.

Dietary restrictions and things to avoid

Food-sensitive eczema reactions typically appear within 6 to 24 hours after an individual consumes a certain food. These reactions can take much longer in some cases.

An elimination diet is often recommended by doctors to decide the foods could be causing the reaction. This diet includes eliminating some of the more popular eczema-causing ingredients.

Before removing any foods, a person should gradually introduce each food category into their diet and monitor their eczema for 4 to 6 weeks to see if they are allergic to any of them.

If a person's symptoms worsen after introducing a new food to their diet, they may choose to stop it in the future. If a person's conditions do not change after removing a food from their diet, they usually do not need to do so.

The following are several popular foods that can cause an eczema flare-up and should be avoided:

- Dairy
- Eggs
- Wheat and/or gluten
- Soy
- Citrus fruits
- Certain spices like cinnamon, cloves and vanilla

- Tomatoes
- Certain nuts

Allergy tests can also be strongly advised by a doctor. Even if a person is not allergic to a food, they may be sensitive to it and develop skin symptoms if they are exposed to it repeatedly. This form of eczema is known as food sensitive eczema by doctors.

People with dyshidrotic eczema, which usually affects the hands and feet, can benefit from avoiding nickel-containing foods. Nickel can be used in trace quantities in the soil and, as a result, in foods.

The following foods are high in nickel:

- Soybeans
- Shellfish
- Seeds
- Nuts

- Beans
- Black tea
- Canned meats
- Chocolate
- Peas
- Lentils

People with eczema are more susceptible to oral allergy syndrome, so if they have a pollen allergy or have moderate allergic reactions to the foods mentioned above, they should see their doctor.

Oral allergy syndrome or susceptibility to birch pollen affects certain individuals with eczema. This suggests they may have adverse reactions to other foods, such as:

- Carrots
- Celiery
- Green apples
- Hazelnuts
- Pears

Most Beneficial Foods for Eczema

While there is no one-size-fits-all eczema diet, consuming a diet high in antioxidants can help alleviate symptoms. Eczema sufferers are prescribed an antioxidant-rich diet that helps to alleviate the condition's symptoms.

A dermatologist will prescribe an eczema diet meal plan tailored to your individual eczema symptoms.

Diets rich in prebiotic foods support the gut microbiome. Prebiotic foods contain fiber that is immune to digestion in the stomach, so bacteria in the intestine ferment them instead. This promotes the growth of beneficial bacteria in the intestine. Fruits, vegetables, and whole grains are all high in fiber.

If you have Eczema, your Eczema meal plan can involve establishing strict eating habits or avoiding a few foods if you are allergic to them.

The Mediterranean Diet

This diet emphasizes the following foods:

- Fish
- Healthy fats
- Olive oil
- Fruits
- Vegetables

It also contains red wine, which contains the antioxidant quercetin. In this diet, sugary sweets and red meat can be consumed in limited amounts or not at all.

The Anti-Inflammatory Diet

This diet focuses on avoiding foods that cause inflammation and consuming foods that are high in fiber. It emphasizes the following:

- Healthy fats
- Olive oil
- Omega-3 fatty acids, found in fish
- Whole grains
- Vegetables
- Fruit
- Chia seeds/pumpkin seeds/flax seeds

Processed foods that are high in chemicals should never be used in this diet.

Cruciferous Vegetables

Broccoli, cauliflower, bok choy, cabbage, garden cress, brussels sprouts, and related vegetables in the Brassicaceae family are high in antioxidants, vitamins, minerals, Omega fatty acids, phytonutrients, carotenoids, and flavonoids.

These vegetables aid in the management of eczema symptoms by reducing inflammation. Furthermore, the high fiber content of these cruciferous foods helps in the removal of toxins from the body, making them an essential food for eczema treatment.

Leafy Greens

Apart from cruciferous vegetables, other green leafy vegetables such as parsley, oregano, and others are high in minerals, flavonoids, and vitamins that help minimize inflammation. Their high enzyme and nutrient content has digestive and restorative properties.

This category of foods improves a person's overall health by strengthening their immune system and supplying adequate nourishment to their body cells, resulting in improved skin health.

Beets

The following are some of the advantages of including beetroot in your eczema diet meal plan:

1. Aids in the repair of damaged cells

2. Red blood cell output is boosted.

3. Aids in the restoration of vital minerals and anti-inflammatory carotenoids.

4. Reintroduces unique enzymes that stimulate glutathione production.

5. Induces the development of inflammatory skin conditions.

Beets are also high in fiber, Vitamin C, antioxidants, and betalains, which are phytonutrients. Betalains are thought to be the best sources for body detoxification and provide superior anti-inflammatory support.

Berries

The antioxidant flavonoid quercetin is abundant in the berry family, which includes blueberries, blackberries, cherries, raspberries, strawberries, cranberries, and others. Antioxidants play a critical role in preventing the onset of diseases and cell damage. The color of the berries has its own meaning when it comes to the nutritious components they contain. These ingredients can help to reduce inflammation.

In addition to the skin benefits, berries are a fruit rich in vitamins and minerals that can help eczema sufferers nourish their bodies. The fruit's fiber content assists in the maintenance of a balanced gut and the elimination of toxins from the body.

Apples

Apples have been found to be one of the most effective foods for skin conditions such as eczema. The fruit acts as a first line of protection against diseases and inflammation. Apples contain a variety of beneficial nutrients such as quercetin, minerals, vitamins, pectin, and phytochemicals, which help to strengthen the immune system, detoxify the body, reduce eczema-related inflammation, and promote rapid healing.

Chicken & Beef Broths

Meat broth is high in the amino acid glycine, which helps to heal skin that has been affected by Atopic Dermatitis. Furthermore, the food is beneficial to the digestive system and eczema. The broth's mineral, amino acid, and collagen content aids in the healing of skin inflammation while not impairing the digestive system.

To achieve the highest consistency, the broth should be cooked on low heat for a longer period of time. The addition of Apple Cider Vinegar is thought to aid in the full removal of nutrients from the meat.

Manuka Honey

Manuka honey has been used as a substitute for safe and radiant skin for a number of years. Its anti-inflammatory properties help to alleviate eczema symptoms and prevent them from worsening. This medicinal honey is said to have a high concentration of enzymes, making it an effective antibacterial agent.

This property aids in the relief of itchiness caused by eczema. Because of its high concentration of Vitamin B, minerals, and amino acids, manuka honey is an excellent food for both internal and external medicinal use.

Turmeric

Curcumin, the herb's main ingredient, is a potential antibacterial and anti-inflammatory agent. As a consequence, turmeric is widely used to relieve eczema-related inflammation. Turmeric contains a large amount of beneficial minerals, fiber, and Vitamin B6, and as a result, it is used as a curative food and aids in the reduction of the immune response caused by eczema.

Papaya

This low-sugar fruit is high in both lycopene and papain, which work together to serve as a powerful antioxidant and aid digestion.

Papaya is important for the following bodily functions:

1. Enhances the regeneration of skin cells
2. Strengthens the immune system
3. It has anti-inflammatory properties.
4. Papaya skin and seeds, in addition to the pulp, are thought to have medicinal and nutritional benefits in the case of eczema by encouraging good digestion.

Food that has been fermented can help with eczema

By adding friendly bacteria into the body, fermented foods can help to strengthen the gut microbiome. While studies on probiotics for eczema have yielded mixed results, allergy researchers are increasingly convinced that probiotics and probiotic-containing foods can help reduce atopic disease in the Western world.

Adults who consume fermented foods have a lower risk of developing eczema. Researchers discovered that mothers who consume more yogurt and fermented foods during pregnancy have a lower chance of their babies developing eczema.

Some examples of fermented foods are:

- Yogurt (natural yogurts)
- Water or milk kefir
- Apple cider vinegar
- Kombucha
- Fermented grains
- Beetroot
- Sauerkraut

Importance of Taking Vitamins

Getting a healthy mix of vitamins, nutrients, and flavonoids in your diet will improve the condition of your skin. **The vitamins and minerals mentioned below are especially important for eczema:**

- Zinc is a mineral that can be used in fish, pumpkin seeds, dark chocolate, and lean red meat.

- Vitamin C is present in vividly colored fruits and vegetables, as well as rosehips.

- Sunflower seeds, almonds, pine nuts, mango, and dried apricots are all high in vitamin E.

- In the summer, Vitamin D is consumed by sunshine. Over the winter, you should even take vitamin D supplements.

- Omega-3's (fatty acids) are found in flaxseed, chia, fatty fish, and other foods. These have anti-inflammatory and heart-protective properties.

- Vitamin K can be found in leafy green vegetables and helps with blood clotting.

Eczema Treatments

1. **Vitamin D Therapy** - Supplementing with vitamin D-rich foods including cod liver oil, sardines, salmon, eggs, and raw milk, in addition to enhancing sun exposure, can help prevent eczema in children and adolescents. Ideally, you can get 2,000-5,000 IU a day during a flare; if your sun exposure is poor, consider supplementing with a high-quality supplement. Low vitamin D levels during pregnancy and childhood may increase the risk of developing eczema, according to preliminary reports.

2. **Compresses that are Cool and Wet** - Some people with eczema find that applying a cold, wet compress relieves their itching. Wet compresses may provide overnight relief from scratching for young children; however, if the eczema has progressed to oozing blisters, a wet compress may raise the risk of infection and should not be used.

3. **Using an anti-itch Cream** - The worst part of an
    eczema flare is usually the constant itching. To get
    much-needed relief, try using a natural homemade
    eczema cream made with Shea butter, coconut oil,
    raw honey, and essential oils.

4. **Phototherapy (also known as light therapy)** -
    Phototherapy, according to the National Eczema
    Association, helps to relieve itching, reduce
    inflammation, improve vitamin D intake, and combat
    bacteria on the skin. Increasing sun exposure by 10–
    15 minutes per day, particularly during an eczema
    flare, will provide relaxation and possibly speed
    healing.

5. **Importance of Moisturizing** - Since dry skin is both a
    cause and a symptom, moisturizing infected areas at
    least twice a day is important. Eczema sufferers would
    love coconut oil as a moisturizer. This antibacterial
    and antifungal eczema treatment has antimicrobial
    properties that offer calming relief and can pace
    healing.

6. **Taking Baths in Dead Sea Salt** - The Dead Sea is known for its soothing properties, and researchers have discovered that bathing in Dead Sea water with salt increases skin hydration, improves skin barrier strength, reduces inflammation, and reduces redness and roughness. (7) Because eczema flare-ups can be exacerbated by extremes of temperature, bath water should be only warm enough to avoid a freeze. Pat the skin dry softly with a fluffy towel rather than rubbing it dry.

7. **Extract of Licorice** - It has been shown in eczema trials that licorice root extract appeared to reduce itching when applied topically. For best performance, mix a few drops with coconut oil or organic itch creams.

8. **Lavender Essential Oils** - Eczema usually induces nausea, sadness, agitation, and inadequate sleep, in addition to the constant itching. Lavender essential oil is a known eczema remedy that can help heal dry skin by reducing these common symptoms. 10 drops of essential oil to 1 tablespoon coconut or almond oil, softly massaged onto the skin when scratching is at its

worst, the scent will also make you sleep better when you're fighting the urge to scratch.

9. **Using Witch Hazel** - Because of its anti-inflammatory and antioxidant effects, witch hazel can help facilitate recovery if the rash appears to ooze after a flare. In a double-blind experiment, researchers discovered that a cream containing witch hazel and phosphatidylcholine can be as powerful as hydrocortisone. Apply this eczema remedy straight to the rash using a cotton pad during an epidemic. If you don't want to induce more dryness, use an alcohol-free witch hazel.

10. **Taking a Vitamin E Supplement** - When dealing with inflammation, taking 400IU of vitamin E daily will help to speed up healing. In addition, applying vitamin E topically will help to alleviate itching and avoid scarring.

11. **Benefits of Goat's Milk Soap** - The use of goat's milk soap as an eczema cure hasn't been thoroughly investigated. However, it does have many advantages

that have been proven to help with eczema therapy.

- Goat's milk soap is a natural exfoliant and it contains lactic acid. Lactic acid, a naturally occurring and gentle alpha-hydroxy acid, is used in goat's milk (AHA). Because of how good it is at exfoliating and promoting cell turnover, lactic acid is still used in some commercial-grade skin peels. Using goat milk soap to cleanse your skin will help remove dead skin cells, exposing new, younger skin cells underneath.

- Probiotics can be found in goat milk's lactic acid. Oral probiotics containing lactic acid bacteria have been found to aid children with eczema. It's worth a shot that these probiotics present in the lactic acid found in goat mllk were an important topical therapy in children.

- Lactic acid does more than just exfoliate the skin and apply probiotics. Lactic acid in goat's milk acts as a natural humectant when mixed with the milk's natural fats and oils. As a result, goat's milk soap can help to reinforce your skin's barrier and lock in moisture. Well-hydrated skin may be less prone to eczema flare-ups.

12.   **Using Pure Aloe Vera Gel** - Aloe vera gel is made from the aloe plant's leaves. Aloe vera gel has been used to treat a variety of illnesses for decades. Eczema relief is a popular use. The benefits of aloe vera gel was researched and found to be antibacterial, antimicrobial, wound healing and immune system boosting. Antibacterial and antimicrobial properties can help avoid skin infections, which are more common in people with dry, broken skin. Aloe's wound-healing properties can help to soothe and heal broken skin. You can buy aloe vera gel in stores or buy aloe plants and use the gel directly from the leaves and applying to the skin.

13.   **Apple Cider Vinegar** - Apple cider vinegar is a well-known home remedy for a variety of ailments, including skin problems, as it helps balance the skin's acidity levels. Vinegar has a high acidity level. The skin is

normally acidic, although eczema patients' skin can be less acidic than others. The skin's defenses can be weakened as a result of this.

Applying diluted apple cider vinegar to the skin may help balance the acidity levels, but if the vinegar is not diluted, it can cause burns.

Many soaps, detergents, and cleansers, on the other hand, are alkaline. They can cause the skin's acidity to be disrupted, leaving it vulnerable to injury. This may explain why some soaps can aggravate eczema flare-ups. Apple cider vinegar has been shown to fight bacteria such as Escherichia coli and Staphylococcus aureus in studies. Using apple cider vinegar on the skin can help prevent infected broken skin.

Before adding apple cider vinegar to the skin, make sure it's diluted. Vinegar that has not been diluted can cause chemical burns or other injuries.

The vinegar can be used in wet wraps or baths, and it can be found in most supermarkets and health food stores.

14.   **Tea-Tree Oil** - The leaves of the Melaleuca alternifolia tree are used to make tea tree oil. This oil is often used to treat skin conditions such as eczema. The oil has anti-inflammatory, antibacterial and wound-healing powers. It can aid in the relief of skin dryness and itching, as well as the prevention of infections.

What to do with it - Before applying essential oils to the skin, always dilute them. Mix tea tree oil with a carrier oil, such as almond or olive oil, and add the mixture. Tea tree oil in a diluted form is used in certain goods.

Home-Made Remedies For Eczema Relief

1. Aloe Vera and Avocado Mask

This mask can be applied to the face to lessen eczema symptoms, or it can be used as a paste to treat other eczema-affected areas of the body. 1 avocado (mashed) a teaspoon of aloe vera gel In a small mixing bowl, combine all of the ingredients. Apply to the face or other parts of the body with a cotton swab. Leave on for 20 minutes before rinsing with warm water. Pat the skin dry.

2. Moisturizer with Coconut Oil

The shelf life of this pure and simple coconut oil moisturizer is pretty long. Make a full batch and use it as your primary facial and body moisturizer as required. 1 cup coconut oil (unrefined) Calendula essential oil, two drops In a pan, combine all of the ingredients. Apply as a daily moisturizer to your face and body. When not in use, keep the coconut oil moisturizer in a container.

3. Soak In An Oatmeal Bath

Fill a nut-milk bag halfway with oats, or place oats in cheesecloth and tie the top shut with a rubber band or string. To make this, use one cup of certified gluten-free rolled oats and one nut-milk bag or cheesecloth. By floating the bag in your bath and gently scrubbing your entire body with it, you can create a relaxing oatmeal bath soak.

4. Salve Made From Olive Leaves

Apply this olive leaf salve during the day or evening to eczema that requires more time to heal, and keep the area covered with gloves or clothes. Mix together a ½ cup of pure shea butter with 2 drops olive leaf extract and store in a tightly sealed jar. Apply this olive leaf salve during the day or evening to eczema that requires more time to heal. Keep the area covered with gloves or clothes for a more intense healing treatment.

5. Apricot Kernel Oil Moisturizing Cream

Mix together a ½ cup of unrefined cocoa butter, ½ cup of unrefined apricot kernel oil and ¼ cup of unrefined neem oil. Combine all ingredients and mix with a blender, food processor or hand mixer. Store in a sealed jar until ready to use. This gentle healing cream can be used on the face or the body. It has a light fragrance from the natural ingredients and a silky smooth texture. Since this is all natural, you can use as much as needed and as often as needed.

6. Olive Oil mixed with Lavender EO

Make an all natural massage oil with olive oil and lavender essential oil. Mix together 1 cup of unrefined olive oil and 2 drops of lavender essential oil. Lavender has a calming effect on the soul, and it also has a calming effect on the physical body. Before going to bed, rub a generous amount of this olive oil and lavender massage oil on the affected areas, or your whole body.

7. Soap Made With Avocado Oil

Starting with a totally pure and plant-based soap bar is the secret to having a gentle liquid soap from this recipe. Look for one that is made entirely of natural ingredients, such as coconut oil, hemp, or another vegetable oil.

You will need (1) 4 oz bar of natural soap, One-gallon of water and ½ cup of unrefined avocado oil. Using a cheese grater, grate the whole soap bar. Remove from the bowl and set aside.

Bring a pot of water to a rolling boil. Remove the pan from the stove and then place the grated soap into the hot water and let sit for 15 minutes, until the soap is completely dissolved.

Next, using a hand mixer, blend the mixture together until you get a smooth consistency. Continue to blend for another minute after adding the avocado oil. Allow time for cooling. To use, pour into a jar with a pump. You just made a wonderful, natural soap for your skin.

8. Make a Natural & Gentle Face Cleanser

To make your own, all natural and gentle face cleanser, which will be soothing and excellent for inflammation, mix together 1 tablespoon of raw honey, 1 tablespoon of yogurt (either coconut milk or plain soy works) and 1 teaspoon of dry and powdered slippery elm.

Combine the ingredients in a bowl and apply all over the face and neck. For twenty seconds, gently rub the entire face in circular motions. After rinsing with warm water, pat dry.

9. Make a Lovely, Turmeric Tea

This eczema recipe begins by balancing the body on the inside so that you can benefit from external healing. You will need 2 filtered cups of water, 1 teaspoon of turmeric powder, 1 teaspoon of raw honey and 1 lemon slice. Once you get your water to a low boil, add your tumeric and let it sit for five to ten minutes for the turmeric to steep. Toss in a pinch of honey and a squeeze of lemon, to taste. Take pleasure in it.

10. Tea with Stinging Nettles

Because healing takes place on the inside, this stinging nettle tea serves a dual purpose when ingested daily and used as a soothing topical treatment for the skin. To make this tea, you will need 4 cups of filtered water, 4 tbsp of raw, unfiltered honey and 4 tbsp of stinging nettle leaves. Get the water to a low boil. Let sit for five to ten minutes of steeping with stinging nettle leaves. Honey should be added at this stage. Drink a cup of the tea every day, and soak a washcloth in the leftover tea to add to the infected areas every day. There's no need to rinse.

11. Magnesium Spray of Sea Salt

I've discovered that drying wet/oozing eczema works easier than attempting to moisturize it. I've always heard people with skin issues say that going to the beach made them feel healthier, which makes sense given the vitamin D from the sun and the magnesium and minerals in the saltwater. If you don't live near the ocean, a homemade magnesium salt spray can provide the same relief for your skin.

12. Evening Primrose Oil

The evening primrose plant produces evening primrose oil. It's a topical treatment for irritated skin. It's used to treat autoimmune inflammatory disorders including eczema as swallowed by mouth. Evening primrose oil is high in omega-6 fatty acids and gamma-linolenic acid, all of which can help to reduce inflammation in the body. Evening primrose oil for eczema has mixed findings in research. Despite this, many people believe that it relieves their eczema symptoms without causing any harmful side effects.

13. Benefits of Sunflower Oil

Sunflower seeds are used to make sunflower oil. It covers the skin's outer layer, which helps hold moisture in and bacteria out, according to research from Trusted Source. Sunflower oil hydrates the skin while also reducing itching and inflammation. Sunflower oil should be added to the skin undiluted, usually after a bath when the skin is still moist.

14. Benefits of Calendula Cream

Calendula cream is a form of herbal medicine. Calendula
has been used as a folk medicine for skin irritation,
wounds, and cuts for decades.

It's believed to assist with blood supply to places of pain
or inflammation, hydration, and infection. Calendula's
potency for eczema is yet to be shown. However, others
argue that it is beneficial.

15. Treating Eczema with Acupuncture & Acupressure

Acupuncture is a technique that involves inserting fine
needles into various points on the body to adjust the flow
of energy. While further research is required, some
studies suggest that acupuncture may help with itching.

Acupressure is similar to acupuncture, but instead of
needles, it uses the fingertips and palms to apply
pressure. preliminary investigation According to Trusted
Source, acupressure can help with itchy skin caused by
eczema.

16. Relaxation Methods

Stress is a frequent cause of eczema flare-ups. Stress is thought to play a role in the development of inflammation, but the precise reason is unknown.

Eczema flare-ups can be reduced by learning to deal with difficult conditions using coping strategies.

Techniques for relaxation that can be beneficial include:

- Deep breathing
- Meditation
- Yoga
- Tai Chi
- Visualization
- Cognitive therapy
- Hypnosis
- Music therapy

Products and Things to Avoid

When dealing with eczema, it's important to avoid and/or eliminate something that might irritate or dry out your skin and cause a flare-up. Items that might trigger your eczema are:

- Pollen
- Body washes or soap with added fragrance
- Any soap or product with dyes/food coloring
- Tight clothes
- Wool clothing
- Animal dander
- Scented laundry products (detergent, softener, dryer sheets, etc)

Things to Keep in Mind

Eczema is a skin disease that can cause significant pain, sleep disturbances, anxiety and depression, as well as skin infections. The number of patients with eczema still have Staphylococcus aureus bacteria on their skin, according to the Mayo Clinic. (13) Serious infections from bacteria and viruses may occur if the rash weeps or if prolonged itching cuts the skin.

Eczema can increase the risk of heart disease and stroke, according to Harvard Medical School study. Eczema patients are more likely to smoke, drink, and exercise than non-eczema patients, according to the report. All three of these causes are linked to an increased risk of heart failure and other chronic illnesses.

During an eczema flare, anxiety, depression, and low sleep quality are real risks for both children and adults. Basic oils for eczema should be diffused or added to lotions or creams to help ease the physical toll that this disease takes on those who suffer from it.

During an epidemic, children are especially vulnerable to ridicule at school, especially if they have eczema on their faces. Children with eczema also withdraw from their social circle and feel alienated. And sure to have lots of patience and encouragement.

If you're suffering from eczema and natural treatment or remedies don't seem to be helping, you should definitely get treatment from a dermatologist.

Also, consult a doctor if you're hoping to get pregnant and have a family history of eczema. They will discuss any precautions you can take to minimize your baby's chances of contracting the disease. Probiotics taken daily by mothers during pregnancy and breastfeeding can help to prevent eczema in their infants.

Conclusion

Although the exact cause of eczema is unknown, contamination, in combination with genetic inheritance, has been shown to have a significant impact on our immune system, which manifests itself in our skin. If you have eczema, there are a variety of options for managing your symptoms and preventing flare-ups. Having a skin care regimen that works for you and sticking to it is the secret. This may include things such as:

Eczema symptoms can be triggered by a variety of factors, like what you eat. While there is no one diet that can cure eczema for anyone, a strong rule of thumb is to avoid any foods that make the symptoms worse. Can you notice that your symptoms worsen when you wear certain clothes, get sweaty, or consume certain foods? Listen to your body about what makes you feel uneasy and want to get away from it as much as possible.

Concentrate on a nutritious diet rich in organic fruits and vegetables, healthy fats, and lean protein. This could help you avoid any, if not all, of your eczema flare-ups.

Most eczema patients benefit by limiting their exposure to environmental allergens, harsh soaps, detergents, and abrupt temperature changes, as well as lowering their stress levels.

Continuous hydration and omega-3 and omega-6 supplementation are the favored solutions for those looking for the more natural eczema treatments. Recent scientific evidence appears to support the belief that omega-3 and omega-6 fatty acids can effectively treat eczema.

Showers and baths should last no longer than 15 minutes, and mild water should be used instead of steam. Instead of rubbing the skin off, pat it off with a towel and moisturize as soon as possible. To seal in moisture and secure your skin's fragile membrane, massage a thick ointment or cream onto your skin at least twice a day, ideally right after bathing.

Use gentle, soap-free cleansers without dyes or perfumes and if you notice anything that is irritating or causing a flare-up, just get rid of it..